Osteoarthritis–Free Hands

5 minutes pain-free exercises to treat your own hand, wrist, Thumb and fingers.

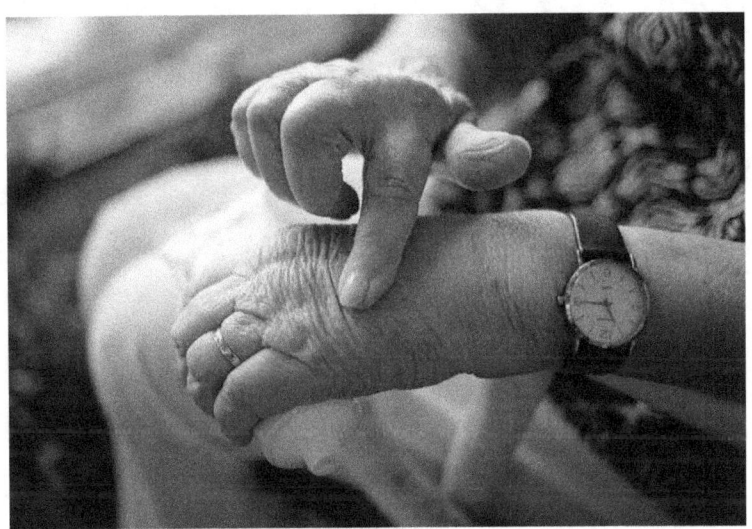

DR. KADEN WINTON

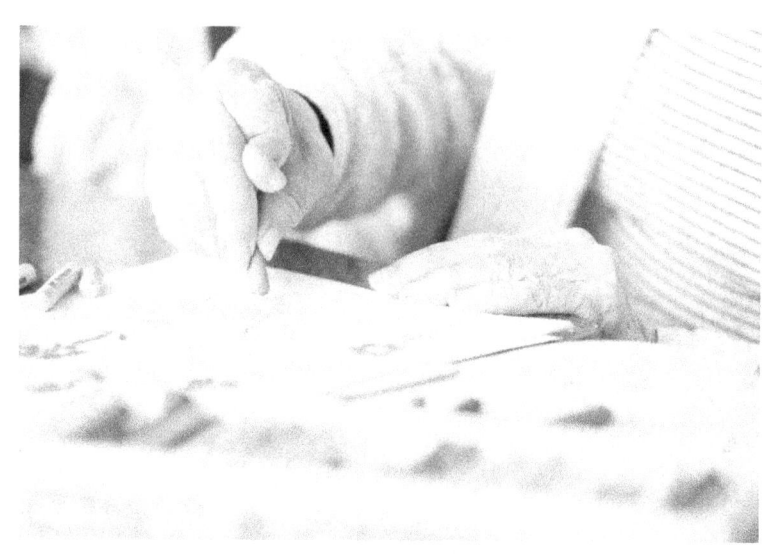

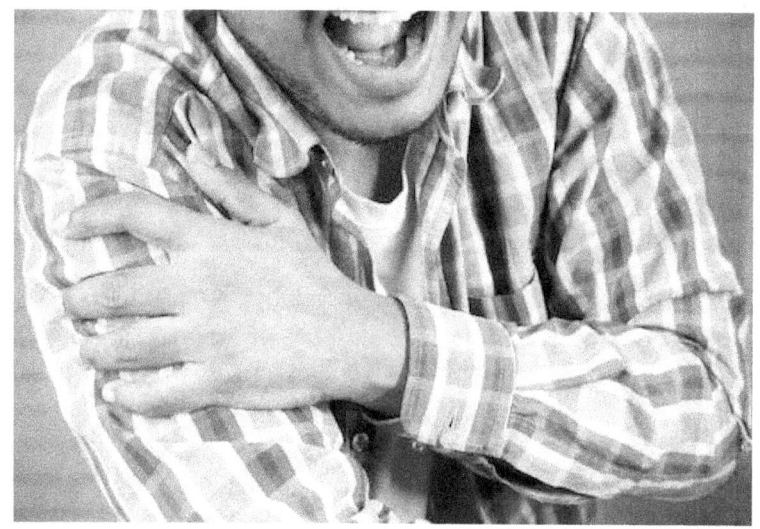

2 | OSTEOARTHRITIS-FREE HAND

Would you like to get deeper insights about this book, or do you have questions that may arise from using this book: kindly send a mail to us @ wintonconsults@gmail.com

Table of Contents

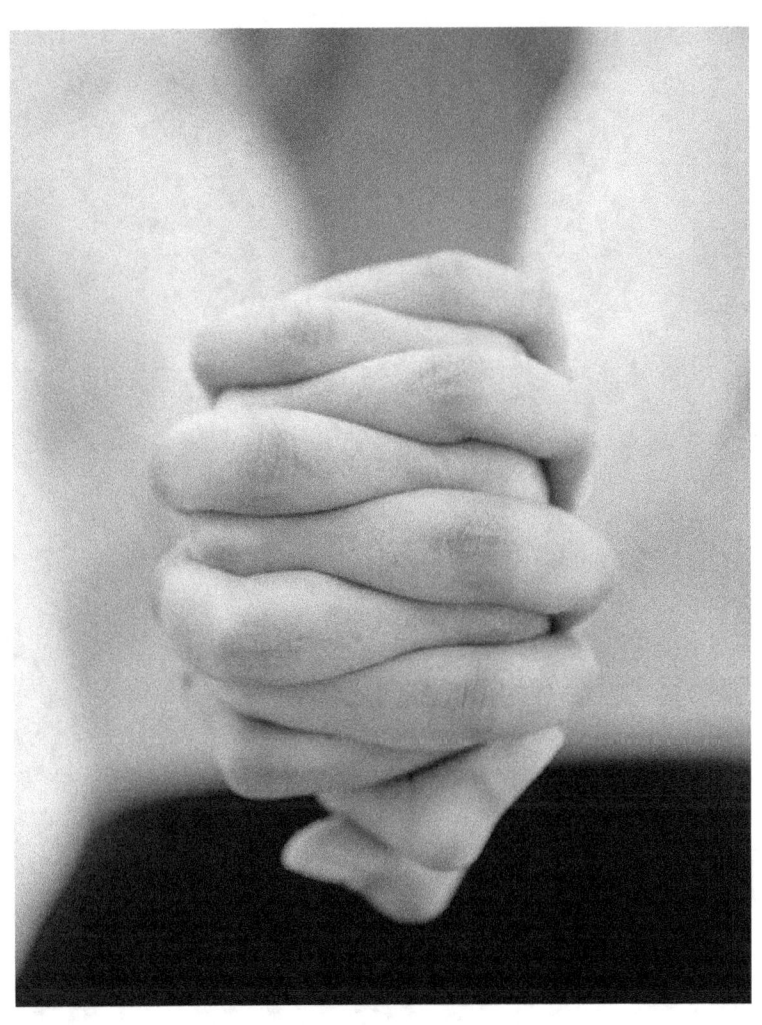

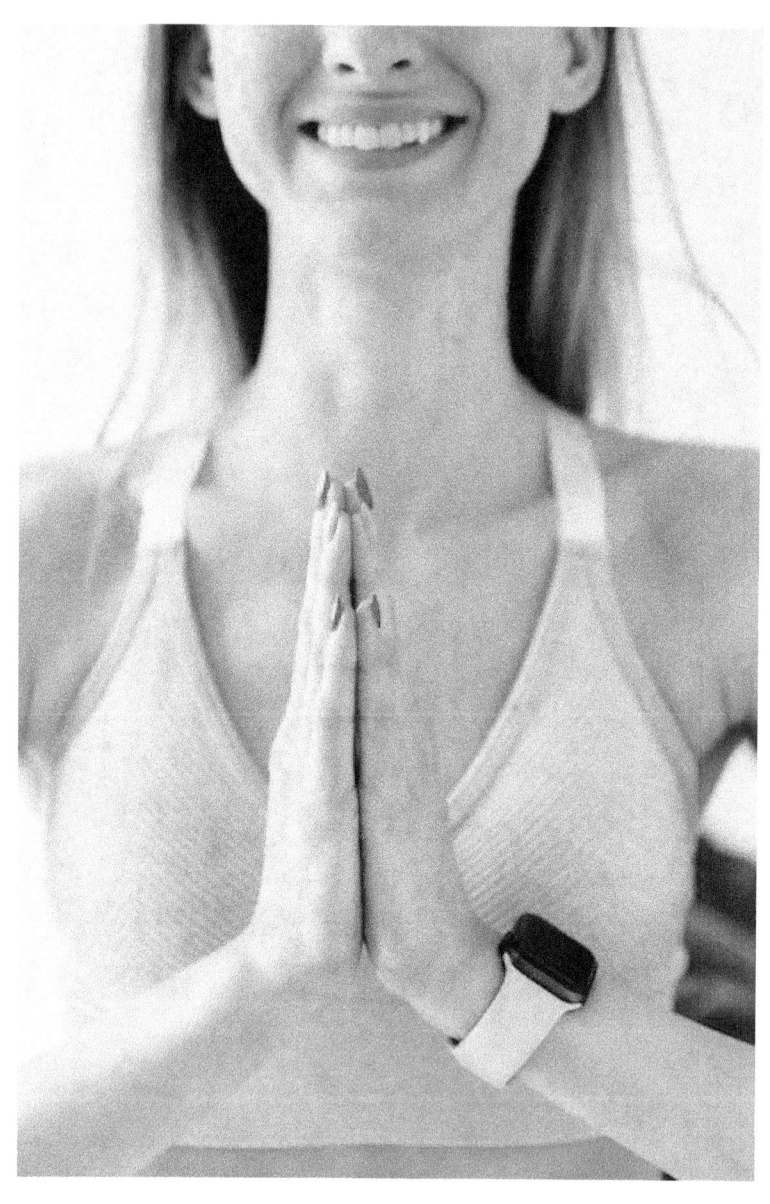

Introduction

A remarkable woman named Margaret lived in a small town nestled amidst rolling hills. Widowed at a young age, Margaret had dedicated her life to raising her four children with unwavering love and a fierce determination to provide for their needs.

Margaret possessed a unique talent—a gift for sewing and creating exquisite dresses that captured the essence of elegance. Her creations were sought after by women far and wide, and her reputation as a skilled seamstress spread like wildfire. Her hands moved swiftly and gracefully, fashioning delicate fabrics into works of art that adorned countless women on special occasions.

As the sole breadwinner, Margaret's nimble fingers were her greatest asset, allowing her to support her family with pride and dignity. The townsfolk admired her for her craftsmanship, resilience, and dedication to her children.

Margaret became an inspiration, a beacon of strength in their close-knit community.

However, fate has a way of testing even the strongest souls. One fateful day, Margaret woke up to an excruciating pain in her hands. Initially dismissing it as a temporary strain from her meticulous work, she continued sewing, pushing through the discomfort. But the pain persisted, intensifying day by day until it became unbearable.

The townspeople noticed the change in Margaret. Her once effortless movements became labored; her smile masked her agony. As her hands stiffened and swelled, she found it increasingly challenging to hold a needle or grasp fabrics with the same precision. Her beloved craft, her lifeline, was now slipping from her grasp.

Visiting the local physician, Margaret was diagnosed with hand osteoarthritis, which threatened to rob her of her livelihood and a sense of purpose. Her heart sank as she realized the implications—the mounting medical bills, the dwindling income, and the inability to provide for her children's needs.

Days turned into weeks, and frustration grew like a storm within Margaret's heart. She tried various remedies, seeking relief from the relentless pain that tormented her. Countless nights were spent in tears, her dreams of a better future shattering like fragile glass.

One gloomy afternoon, as Margaret wandered through the town, her eyes were drawn to a small, inviting bookshop. She stepped inside, her wearied soul seeking solace within the pages of literature. A glimmer of hope caught her eye among the rows of books—an unassuming book titled "Osteoarthritis-Free Hands: 5-Minute Easy Exercises to Treat Your Hand, Wrist, and Fingers."

Intrigued, Margaret delicately picked up the book, her fingers caressing the worn pages. With a flicker of hope, she began reading the words that promised relief from her relentless pain. The exercises described within its chapters seemed simple yet effective, offering a chance to regain control over her life.

With renewed determination, Margaret immersed herself in the book's teachings. Every day, despite the pain and stiffness, she diligently practised the exercises, devoting five precious minutes to the well-being of her hands. It was not an easy journey—there were moments of doubt, frustration, and setbacks—but Margaret persevered, fueled by her love for her children and the yearning to regain her independence.

As the weeks passed, Margaret noticed a gradual improvement. The pain subsided, the swelling diminished, and her once-stiff joints began to loosen. With each passing day, her hands regained their agility and strength, and a glimmer of hope bloomed within her heart once more.

One sunny morning, Margaret triumphantly picked up a piece of fabric, her hands gliding effortlessly across its surface. She stitched with a renewed passion, creating a dress that radiated beauty and resilience—a symbol of her triumph over adversity.

Word of Margaret's return to her craft spread like wildfire through the town. The townsfolk, who had once admired her creations, now marvelled at her resilience and unwavering spirit. Margaret's dresses adorned not only the women of the town but also their hearts, serving as a reminder of the power of determination and the ability to overcome even the greatest challenges.

Margaret's journey restored her ability to provide for her children and gifted her with a newfound purpose—to share her story, her struggles, and the exercises that had relieved her. With her heart overflowing with gratitude, Margaret vowed to help others battling hand osteoarthritis, offering them a beacon of hope in their darkest moments.

And so, Margaret's legacy extended beyond her exquisite dresses, weaving a tapestry of resilience, hope, and the transformative power of self-care. Her story became an inspiration, reminding all who heard it that with perseverance and the right tools, one could conquer the greatest trials and emerge stronger on the other side.

In the realm of battling osteoarthritis, where every movement can be a daunting task, a glimmer of hope emerges from the pages of this book. Within its essence lies a collection of transformative exercises, carefully curated to alleviate the burdensome pain and limitations caused by hand osteoarthritis.

For those grappling with this debilitating condition, the simple yet powerful exercises presented within these chapters hold the key to reclaiming a life of freedom and renewed vitality. With each turn of the page, a path towards relief unfolds, a promising respite from the relentless grip of osteoarthritis.

Gone are the days of resigned acceptance and overwhelming frustration. Embrace the possibility of a brighter future where pain no longer dictates the course of your life. By devoting five minutes a day to these exercises, you can strengthen weakened joints, increase flexibility, and restore a sense of control over your hands.

Allow the knowledge and wisdom within these pages to be your guiding light on this transformative journey. Discover how gentle finger taps, wrist rotations, and thumb stretches can unlock a world of possibilities. You will embark on self-healing and empowerment through meticulously crafted movements.

Join a community of individuals seeking solace from the throes of hand osteoarthritis as they share their stories of triumph and resilience. Let this book be your steadfast companion, providing a comprehensive understanding of the condition and the tools to embrace a life free from the constraints of osteoarthritis.

Together, let us embark on a transformative odyssey as we unlock the power of these five-minute exercises, restoring hope, reclaiming joy, and setting our hands free from the shackles of osteoarthritis.

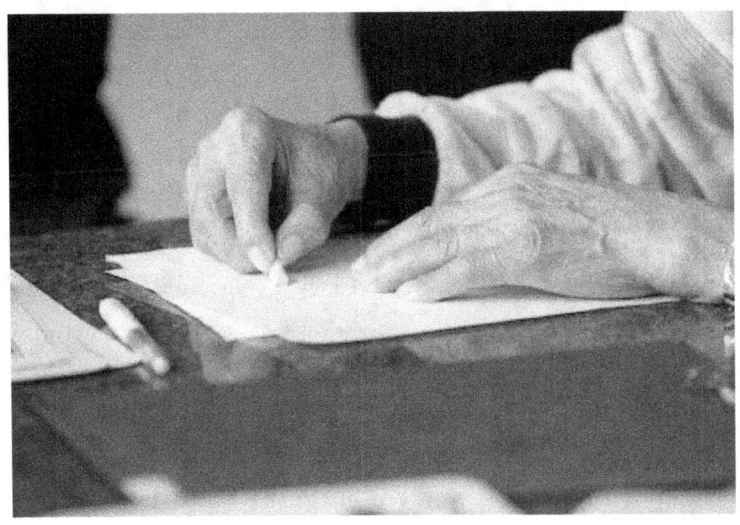

Chapter One

Understanding Osteoarthritis in the Hands

Osteoarthritis is a common degenerative joint disease that affects millions of people worldwide. Hand osteoarthritis is prevalent in various forms and can significantly impact a person's daily life. In this article, we will delve into the intricacies of hand osteoarthritis, exploring its causes, symptoms, and diagnostic methods, to foster a better understanding of this condition.

What is Osteoarthritis?

Osteoarthritis is a chronic condition characterized by the breakdown of cartilage, the protective tissue that cushions the joints. Over time, the cartilage gradually wears away, leading to joint pain, stiffness, and reduced mobility. While osteoarthritis can affect any joint in the body, it frequently manifests in the hands.

How Osteoarthritis Affects the Hands

Hand osteoarthritis primarily affects the joints in the fingers, thumbs, and wrists. The disease commonly develops in the distal interphalangeal joints (DIP), proximal interphalangeal joints (PIP), and the base of the thumb. As the cartilage deteriorates, the affected joints become inflamed, leading to pain, swelling, and a diminished range of motion. Everyday tasks such as gripping objects, opening jars, or even buttoning clothing can become challenging and painful.

Causes and Risk Factors

The exact cause of hand osteoarthritis remains unknown, but several factors contribute to its development. Ageing is a significant risk factor, as joint wear and tear increase the likelihood of cartilage breakdown over time. Other risk factors include genetics, previous hand injuries, repetitive hand motions, obesity, and certain metabolic conditions such as diabetes.

Signs and Symptoms

Hand osteoarthritis presents a range of symptoms that may vary in severity among individuals. Common signs include joint pain, stiffness, and swelling. Morning stiffness, which typically improves within 30 minutes, is a hallmark of osteoarthritis. As the condition progresses, bony nodules called Heberden's nodes may develop on the distal finger joints, and Bouchard's nodes may form on the proximal finger joints. These nodules can be tender to the touch and further limit joint movement.

Do you feel discomfort around your knee simultaneously, you can check up a tailored approach to healing knee osteoarthritis here. For consultations, you can always reach us @ wintonconsults@gmail.com

Diagnosis of Hand Osteoarthritis

Diagnosing hand osteoarthritis involves a thorough assessment of symptoms, a physical examination, and, in some cases, medical imaging. The doctor will inquire about the patient's medical history, including any previous hand injuries or familial predisposition to the disease. During the physical examination, the doctor will examine the affected joints for tenderness, swelling, and signs of nodules. X-rays and other imaging techniques may be used to visualize the joint structure, assess the degree of cartilage loss, and rule out other possible causes of hand pain.

Understanding the nature of hand osteoarthritis is crucial in managing its impact on one's daily life. This degenerative joint condition can significantly hinder hand function and cause chronic pain. By recognizing the signs and symptoms of hand osteoarthritis and seeking an accurate diagnosis, individuals can access appropriate treatment and management strategies to alleviate their symptoms and improve their quality of life.

While hand osteoarthritis is a lifelong condition, various treatment options, including medication, splints, physical therapy, and lifestyle modifications, can help manage pain, reduce inflammation, and maintain hand function. Additionally, staying physically active, maintaining a healthy weight, and protecting the hands from excessive strain or injury can be vital in managing the disease's progression.

In the next chapter of this book, we will evaluate the benefits of exercises to hand health and osteoarthritis healing.

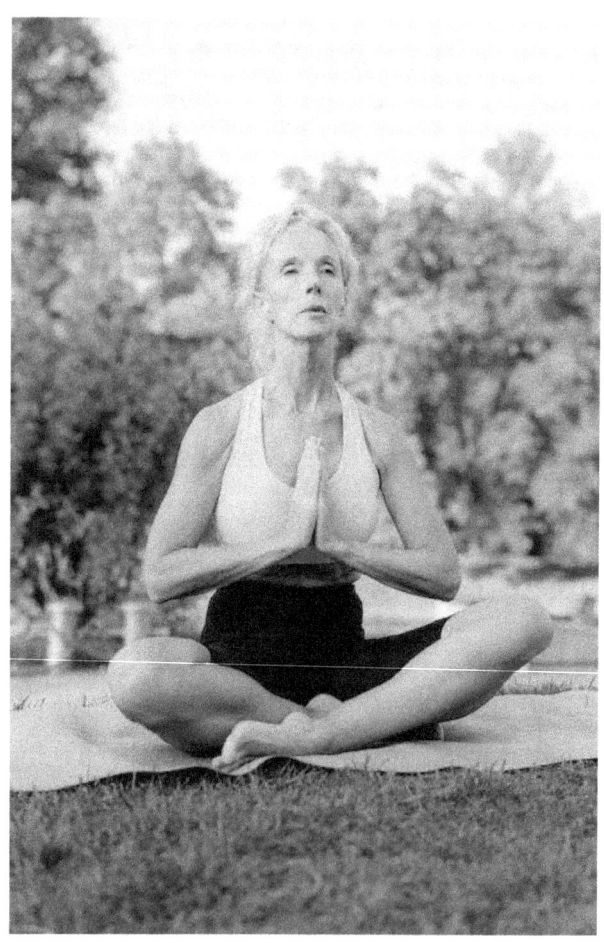

Chapter Two

Unlocking the healing Power of Movement

When managing hand osteoarthritis, exercise is a potent tool that can make a difference. Far from being a burden, regular physical activity tailored to the needs of the hands can offer numerous benefits, from reducing pain and stiffness to enhancing strength, range of motion, flexibility, and agility. In this chapter, we will delve into the significance of exercise in managing hand osteoarthritis and explore its multifaceted advantages.

Benefits of Exercise for Hand Health

Engaging in targeted exercises for hand osteoarthritis provides many benefits that positively impact overall hand health. Exercise helps to increase blood circulation, which promotes the delivery of vital nutrients to the affected joints and aids in removing metabolic waste products. Additionally, exercise supports the health of surrounding tissues, including ligaments, tendons, and muscles, which play a crucial role in hand function.

Role of Exercise in Reducing Pain and Stiffness

One of the most significant advantages of exercise in managing hand osteoarthritis is its ability to alleviate pain and reduce stiffness. Regular physical activity stimulates the production and release of endorphins, the body's natural pain-relieving chemicals, providing a natural anal

gesic effect. Moreover, exercise promotes the production of synovial fluid, which lubricates the joints, reducing friction and stiffness.

Strengthening the Muscles and Joints:

Exercise is a powerful tool for strengthening the muscles and joints affected by hand osteoarthritis. Strengthening exercises target the surrounding muscles, enhancing their ability to support the joints and reducing strain during everyday activities. By improving muscular strength, individuals can experience greater stability and improved hand function, minimizing the impact of osteoarthritis.

Improving Range of Motion:

Hand osteoarthritis often restricts the range of motion, making simple tasks challenging. However, through regular exercise, individuals can improve their range of motion and regain functional abilities. Range-of-motion exercises focus on gently moving the joints through their full range, helping to maintain flexibility and prevent joint stiffness. Over time, consistent practice can lead to noticeable improvements in hand mobility and the ability to perform daily activities more easily.

Enhancing Flexibility and Dexterity:

Flexibility and agility are vital for maintaining optimal hand function. Exercise routines that incorporate stretching and agility exercises can help improve flexibility and fine motor skills. Stretching exercises target the muscles and tendons, increasing their flexibility and reducing the risk of injury. Dexterity exercises, such as finger tapping, squeezing stress balls, and picking up small objects, challenge the coordination and control of the hand, promoting agility and precision.

Incorporating Exercise into the Routine

Before starting an exercise program for hand osteoarthritis, it is essential to consult with a healthcare professional or a qualified hand therapist. They can provide personalized recommendations based on the individual's condition, pain level, and overall health.

Exercise programs for hand osteoarthritis often include a combination of range-of-motion, strengthening, stretching, and dexterity exercises. It is crucial to start slowly and gradually increase the intensity and duration of the exercises as tolerated. Consistency is key, and regular exercise can yield significant benefits over time, even for short periods.

Additionally, individuals should be mindful of their limits and avoid overexertion or activities that exacerbate pain. Applying heat or cold therapy before or after exercise sessions can help manage discomfort. Using assistive devices, such as hand splints or ergonomic tools, can also aid in minimizing strain on the joints during exercises and daily tasks.

Exercise is pivotal in managing hand osteoarthritis, offering a holistic approach to pain relief, increased functionality, and improved quality of life. Through regular exercise, individuals can reduce pain, alleviate stiffness, strengthen muscles and joints, improve range of motion, and enhance flexibility and agility.

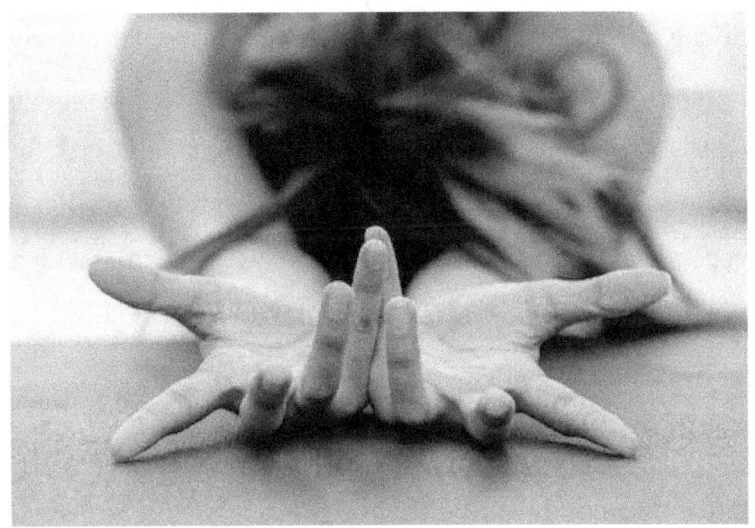

Chapter Three

Getting Started

Embarking on an exercise journey to manage hand osteoarthritis is a commendable decision that promises improved hand function and reduced pain. However, before diving into the exercises, it is crucial to prepare adequately to ensure safety, maximize effectiveness, and maintain consistency. This article will explore essential steps for preparing for the exercises, including safety guidelines, necessary equipment, creating an exercise routine, tracking progress, and tips for maintaining consistency.

Safety Guidelines

Safety should always be the top priority when exercising, especially for individuals with hand osteoarthritis. Before starting any exercise program, consulting with a healthcare professional or a qualified hand therapist is essential. They can provide valuable guidance and tailor exercises to suit individual needs, considering factors such as pain level, joint stability, and overall health.

Furthermore, listening to your body and avoiding pushing through excessive pain or discomfort is important. Start with gentle exercises and gradually increase intensity as tolerated. If any exercise exacerbates pain or causes significant discomfort, it is advisable to discontinue that particular movement and seek guidance from a healthcare professional.

Equipment and Accessories

While many exercises for hand osteoarthritis can be performed without specialized equipment, certain tools and accessories can enhance the effectiveness and comfort of the exercise routine. Some examples include:

- Hand therapy or stress balls: These equipment provide resistance and can be squeezed to strengthen hand muscles.

- Hand splints or braces: This support and stabilize the affected joints during exercises and daily activities.

- Grip aids or ergonomic tools: This help reduce hand strain and improve grip during exercises or everyday tasks.

Creating an Exercise Routine

Developing a structured exercise routine is essential for consistent progress and optimal results. Here are a few key considerations:

- Frequency: Aim for regular exercise sessions, ideally several times weekly. Consistency is key to reaping the benefits of the exercises.

- Duration: Start with shorter sessions, gradually increasing the duration as tolerated. Aim for at least 10-15 minutes per session.

- Warm-up and cool-down: Incorporate gentle warm-up exercises to prepare the hands for activity and cool-down stretches to promote flexibility and relaxation.

- Exercise variety: Include a mix of range-of-motion exercises, strengthening exercises, stretching, and dexterity exercises to target different aspects of hand health and function.

- Gradual progression: Gradually increase the intensity or difficulty of exercises over time as strength and flexibility improve.

Tailoring the exercise routine to personal preferences and goals can help maintain motivation and enjoyment.

Tracking Progress and Results

Tracking progress is an important aspect of any exercise program, as it provides motivation and helps evaluate the effectiveness of the exercises. Consider the following methods for tracking progress:

- Keep a journal: Document the exercises performed, the duration, and any notable changes or improvements observed. This can serve as a reference point for future assessments.

- Monitor pain levels: Track pain levels before, during, and after exercise sessions to gauge changes in symptom severity.

- Measure range of motion: Use simple tools, such as a goniometer or visual markers, to measure and track improvements in joint flexibility and range of motion.

- Assess functional abilities: Take note of any improvements in performing daily activities previously challenging due to hand osteoarthritis.

Regularly reviewing progress can provide a sense of accomplishment and highlight the positive impact of the exercises. For this purpose of record keeping, a free exercise tracker is provided at the closing pages of this book to assist you monitor your progress.

Tips for Maintaining Consistency

Consistency is key to achieving long-term benefits from exercise. Consider the following tips to maintain

Motivation and consistency:

- Set realistic goals: Establish attainable goals that are specific, measurable, and time-bound. Breaking larger goals into smaller milestones can provide a sense of achievement.

- Find a supportive community: Joining support groups or connecting with others with similar goals can provide encouragement, advice, and a sense of camaraderie.

- Incorporate exercise into daily routines: Integrate exercises into daily activities, such as watching TV or during designated breaks, to make them a regular part of the day.

- Celebrate successes: Acknowledge and celebrate milestones and achievements, no matter how small. Rewarding oneself can reinforce positive behavior and maintain motivation.

Preparing for exercises is crucial in optimizing the benefits of managing hand osteoarthritis. By adhering to safety guidelines, identifying the necessary equipment, creating a tailored exercise routine, tracking progress, and maintaining consistency, individuals can embark on a successful journey toward improved hand function, reduced pain, and a better quality of life. Remember, preparation is the foundation for success, and with dedication and commitment, the exercises can become a valuable tool in managing hand osteoarthritis effectively.

Chapter Four

The Five-Minute Easy Exercises for Hand, Thumb, Wrist, and Fingers

Regular exercise is vital in managing hand osteoarthritis and incorporating a simple five-minute routine into your daily life can make a significant difference. These easy exercises target the hand, wrist, and fingers, improving strength, flexibility, and range of motion while reducing pain and stiffness. This step-by-step guide will walk you through each exercise, providing detailed instructions to ensure proper technique and maximize the benefits.

Exercise 1: Finger Taps

- Sit comfortably with your forearm supported on a table or your lap.

- Slowly lift one finger at a time, starting with the thumb, then the index finger, middle finger, ring finger, and pinky.

- Lower each finger back to the starting position, tapping the table lightly.

- Repeat this tapping motion for each finger, aiming for 10 taps per finger.

- Increase the speed gradually while maintaining control and precision.

Exercise 2: Wrist Rotations

- Extend your right arm in front of you, palm down.

- Gently rotate your wrist in a circular motion, clockwise and counterclockwise.

- Perform 10 rotations in each direction.

- Focus on keeping the movement smooth and controlled, avoiding sudden or jerky motions.

Exercise 3: Thumb Stretch

- Hold your hand in a relaxed position with your fingers extended.

- Gently bring your thumb across your palm towards the base of your pinky finger, creating a stretch in the thumb.

- Hold the stretch for 10-15 seconds.

- Release and repeat the stretch on the other hand.

- Aim for 3-5 repetitions on each hand, gradually increasing the duration of the stretch over time.

Exercise 4: Grip Strengthener

- Hold a soft stress ball, hand therapy ball, or a similar object in your hand.

- Squeeze the ball with your fingers and thumb, applying moderate pressure.

- Hold the squeeze for 5 seconds and then release.

- Repeat this squeezing motion 10 times, focusing on engaging the muscles in your hand and forearm.

Exercise 5: Finger Flexion and Extension

- Begin with your hand extended and fingers straight.

- Slowly curl your fingers into a fist, bringing the fingertips towards the base of the fingers.

- Hold the fist for a few seconds and gently open your hand, extending your fingers back to the starting position.

- Repeat this flexion and extension motion for 10 repetitions, focusing on smooth and controlled movements.

Exercise 6: Hand Squeezes

- Place a soft stress ball or hand therapy ball in the palm of your hand.

- Squeeze the ball firmly with your fingers and palm, applying steady pressure.

- Hold the squeeze for 5 seconds and then release.

- Repeat the squeezing motion 10 times on each hand, focusing on building hand strength and coordination.

Exercise 7: Wrist Flexion and Extension

- Sit with your forearm supported on a table or your lap.

- Extend your right arm in front of you, palm down.

- Slowly bend your wrist upward, bringing your palm towards the ceiling.

- Hold the stretch for a few seconds and slowly lower your wrist, returning your palm to the starting position.

- Repeat this flexion and extension motion for 10 repetitions, focusing on maintaining a smooth and controlled movement.

Exercise 8: Finger Abduction and Adduction

- Begin with your hand relaxed and your fingers together.

- Slowly spread your fingers apart, creating space between each finger.

- Hold the stretch for a few seconds, then bring your fingers back together.

- Repeat this abduction and adduction motion for 10 repetitions, focusing on gentle and controlled movements.

These five-minute easy exercises for the hand, wrist, and fingers provide a practical and time-efficient approach to managing hand osteoarthritis. By incorporating these exercises into your daily routine, you can improve hand strength, flexibility, and range of motion, while reducing pain and stiffness. Remember to start slowly, listen to your body, and gradually increase intensity as tolerated. Consistency is key, so aim to perform these exercises daily to experience the long-term benefits.

Chapter Five

Exploring Additional Techniques and Therapies in Hand Osteoarthritis Management

In addition to exercise, various techniques and therapies can further support individuals in effectively managing hand osteoarthritis. These additional approaches can complement exercise routines, relieve symptoms, enhance hand function, and improve overall well-being. In this chapter, we will explore a range of techniques and therapies, including heat and cold therapy, assistive devices, hand splints and braces, lifestyle modifications, and complementary and alternative therapies.

Heat and Cold Therapy

Heat and cold therapy are simple yet effective techniques that can help alleviate pain and reduce inflammation in the hands affected by osteoarthritis.

- Heat therapy: Applying heat to the hands can help increase blood flow, relax muscles, and ease stiffness. Options for heat therapy include warm water baths, warm towels or heat packs, or paraffin wax baths. Ensuring the temperature is comfortable and not too hot is important to avoid burns or further discomfort.

- Cold therapy: Cold therapy reduces inflammation and numbing pain. Applying cold packs or ice wrapped in a towel to the affected area can help alleviate swelling and provide temporary relief. Limiting cold therapy sessions to 10-15 minutes is advisable to prevent frostbite or skin damage.

Assistive Devices for Daily Activities

Assistive devices are valuable tools that can support individuals in maintaining independence and performing daily activities with greater ease. These devices are designed to reduce strain on the hands and provide support to weakened joints. Some common assistive devices for hand osteoarthritis include:

- Jar openers and bottle grippers: These aids help open jars, bottles, and containers requiring grip strength.

- Adaptive kitchen utensils: These have larger handles or specialized grips that make them easier to hold and use for cooking and eating.

- Reacher or grabber tools: These devices assist in picking up objects from the floor or reaching items on higher shelves without putting excessive strain on the hands.

- Ergonomic pens and pencils: These writing tools have a design that promotes a more relaxed and comfortable grip.

By incorporating assistive devices into daily routines, individuals can minimize joint stress and continue to perform tasks independently.

Hand Splints and Braces

Hand splints and braces are orthopaedic devices that support, stabilize, and immobilize the affected joints. These devices are particularly beneficial for individuals with significant pain or joint instability. Hand splints and braces can:

- Reduce pain: By limiting the movement of affected joints, splints and braces can help alleviate pain and discomfort.

- Improve joint alignment: These devices assist in maintaining proper joint alignment, which can prevent further deterioration and promote healing.

- Provide support: Hand splints and braces offer external support to weakened or unstable joints, reducing the risk of injury during activities.

It is important to consult with a healthcare professional or hand therapist to determine the appropriate type of splint or brace and ensure proper fitting for optimal benefit.

Lifestyle Modifications in Managing Osteoarthritis

Lifestyle modifications are crucial for managing hand osteoarthritis and promoting overall joint health. Some key lifestyle adjustments include:

- Maintain a healthy weight: Excess weight can increase joint stress, exacerbating hand osteoarthritis symptoms. By maintaining a healthy weight through a balanced diet and regular exercise, individuals can alleviate the strain on their hands.

- Practice joint protection techniques: Learning proper body mechanics and techniques for performing daily activities can minimize joint stress. For example, using larger joints (like the shoulder) instead of smaller joints (like the fingers) to carry heavy loads can reduce strain.

- Take regular breaks: When engaging in activities that require repetitive hand movements

It is important to take regular breaks to rest the hands and reduce the risk of overuse injuries such as typing or crafting.

- Modify the environment: Simple modifications to the home or workplace can help create a more ergonomic environment. Using cushioned mats, adjustable chairs, or supportive wrist pads can alleviate strain on the hands during activities.

Individuals can better manage symptoms and promote hand health by implementing these lifestyle modifications.

Complementary and Alternative Therapies

Complementary and alternative therapies can be considered adjuncts to conventional treatments for hand osteoarthritis. While scientific evidence supporting their effectiveness varies, some individuals find them beneficial in managing symptoms and improving overall well-being. Examples of complementary and alternative therapies include:

- Acupuncture: This traditional Chinese therapy involves the insertion of thin needles into specific points on the body to promote pain relief and balance energy flow.

- Massage therapy: Techniques such as gentle joint mobilization and soft tissue manipulation can help alleviate pain, reduce muscle tension, and improve circulation.

- Herbal supplements: Certain herbal supplements, such as ginger or turmeric, are believed to possess anti-inflammatory properties. However, consulting with a healthcare professional before starting supplements is important to ensure safety and avoid medication interactions.

- Mind-body techniques: Practices like yoga, meditation, and tai chi can help promote relaxation, reduce stress, and improve overall well-being. These techniques may also enhance body awareness and improve joint mobility.

While complementary and alternative therapies can be explored, consulting with a healthcare professional before initiating any new therapies is crucial, especially if you have underlying medical conditions or are taking medications.

By incorporating additional techniques and therapies into your hand osteoarthritis management plan, you can further enhance the effectiveness of exercise and experience greater relief from symptoms. Heat and cold therapy, assistive devices, hand splints and braces, lifestyle modifications, and complementary and alternative therapies offer valuable tools for reducing pain, improving function, and promoting overall well-being.

Chapter Six

Tips for Preventing Hand Osteoarthritis

Additional Techniques and Therapies for Hand Osteoarthritis explored various methods to complement exercise and enhance symptom management. Now, let us delve into an equally important topic: Tips for Preventing Hand Osteoarthritis. By adopting preventive measures and practising proactive habits, individuals can reduce the likelihood of developing this condition and maintain optimal hand health.

Maintaining a Healthy Weight

Maintaining a healthy weight is one of the fundamental pillars of preventing hand osteoarthritis. Excess weight places additional stress on the joints, including those in the hands, accelerating the wear and tear. By adopting a balanced diet and regular exercise, individuals can manage their weight and decrease the risk of developing hand osteoarthritis. It's important to focus on consuming a nutritious diet that includes fruits, vegetables, lean proteins, and whole grains while limiting processed foods, sugary drinks, and saturated fats. Regular physical activity, such as walking, swimming, or cycling, can help promote joint health and overall well-being.

Ergonomic Principles for Hand Care

Incorporating ergonomic principles into daily activities is crucial for minimizing strain on the hands and reducing the risk of developing hand osteoarthritis. By paying attention to ergonomics, individuals can create an environment that supports hand health. Some key tips for practising ergonomic principles include maintaining proper posture, using ergonomic tools and equipment, taking regular breaks, and positioning the hands correctly. These adjustments can alleviate unnecessary strain and promote optimal hand function during activities.

Avoiding Overuse and Repetitive Strain

Overuse and repetitive strain are significant contributors to hand osteoarthritis. By being mindful of these factors and adopting preventive strategies, individuals can protect their hands from unnecessary stress. Taking frequent breaks during repetitive hand activities, alternating tasks to distribute stress, using proper technique and body mechanics, and utilizing assistive devices are effective ways to avoid overuse and minimize the risk of developing hand osteoarthritis.

Protecting the Hands from Injuries

Injuries to the hands can increase the likelihood of developing hand osteoarthritis. Therefore, taking precautions and practising safety measures to protect the hands is crucial. Wearing protective gloves during activities that carry a risk of a hand injury, using proper hand posture during tasks, avoiding repetitive trauma, and being cautious during physical activities are essential steps for safeguarding the hands from injuries that could contribute to hand osteoarthritis.

Incorporating Joint-Friendly Habits

Incorporating joint-friendly habits into daily routines is an excellent way to support hand health and reduce the risk of developing hand osteoarthritis. Some recommended habits include maintaining hand flexibility through regular exercises and stretches, practising good hand hygiene to prevent infections, avoiding excessive force during tasks, and managing stress. By implementing these habits, individuals can prioritize their hands' long-term health and functionality.

By integrating these tips for preventing hand osteoarthritis into your lifestyle, you can take proactive measures to protect your hands and reduce the risk of developing this condition. Remember, prevention is always better than cure. When combined with regular exercise, additional techniques, and therapies discussed earlier, these strategies form a comprehensive approach to hand osteoarthritis management.

Do you feel discomfort around your hip, you can check up a tailored approach to healing hip osteoarthritis here. For consultations, you can always reach us @ wintonconsults@gmail.com

Bonus

The 7- Day Osteoarthritis Meal Plan

It is essential to adopt an anti-inflammatory diet to enhance the effectiveness of the exercises provided in this book and support the management of hand osteoarthritis. Nutrition reduces inflammation, promotes joint health, and supports the body's natural healing processes. By incorporating specific foods and nutrients known for their anti-inflammatory properties, individuals can further optimize their journey towards relieving pain and maintaining healthy hands.

Exercise is a key component of managing hand osteoarthritis, as it helps improve joint mobility, strengthen muscles, and reduce pain and stiffness. The exercises outlined in this book are designed to target the hands, wrists, and fingers, providing relief and enhancing functionality. However, exercise alone is not sufficient to achieve optimal results. Combining exercise with an anti-inflammatory diet can significantly enhance the benefits and improve overall well-being.

An anti-inflammatory diet focuses on consuming foods rich in antioxidants, omega-3 fatty acids, and other nutrients known for their anti-inflammatory properties. These nutrients help combat inflammation, reduce pain, and support joint health. Incorporating fruits, vegetables, whole grains, fatty fish, nuts, and seeds can provide the body with essential nutrients and promote healing from within.

To assist you in implementing an anti-inflammatory diet that complements your exercise routine, we have prepared a 7-day meal plan. Each day offers a variety of nutrient-dense, anti-inflammatory foods to support your hand health and overall well-being. Here is a sample of what the meal plan includes:

Day 1:

- **Breakfast:** Overnight oats with berries and a sprinkle of chia seeds.

- **Lunch:** Grilled salmon with roasted vegetables.

- **Snack:** Fresh fruit salad with a handful of almonds.

- **Dinner:** Quinoa salad with mixed greens, grilled chicken, and avocado.

- **Dessert:** Mixed berry smoothie with a touch of turmeric.

Day 2:

- **Breakfast:** omelette with spinach and mushrooms served with whole-grain toast.

- **Lunch:** Lentil soup with a side of steamed broccoli.

- **Snack:** Greek yogurt with sliced cucumbers and a drizzle of olive oil.

- **Dinner:** Baked cod with quinoa and roasted asparagus.

- **Dessert:** Dark chocolate-covered strawberries.

Day 3:

- **Breakfast:** Eggs scrambled with spinach and tomatoes.

- **Lunch:** Chickpea salad with mixed greens, cherry tomatoes, and feta cheese.

- **Snack:** Carrot sticks with hummus.

- **Dinner:** Chicken breast grilled with quinoa and roasted Brussels sprouts.

- **Dessert:** Mango and pineapple sorbet.

Day 4:

- **Breakfast:** Berry smoothie bowl topped with granola and sliced almonds.

- **Lunch:** Grilled vegetable wrap with whole-grain tortilla.

- **Snack:** Celery sticks with almond butter.

- **Dinner:** Baked tofu with brown rice and steamed bok choy.

- **Dessert:** Chia seed pudding with fresh berries and coconut milk.

Day 5:

- **Breakfast:** Avocado toast with smoked salmon and a squeeze of lemon.

- **Lunch:** Quinoa and black bean salad with diced bell peppers and cilantro.

- **Snack:** Roasted chickpeas.

- **Dinner:** Meatballs made of turkey, served with zucchini noodles and marinara sauce.

- **Dessert:** Mixed berry parfait with Greek yogurt.

Day 6:

- **Breakfast:** Vegetable omelet served with whole-grain toast.

- **Lunch:** Spinach salad with grilled chicken, strawberries, and walnuts.

- **Snack:** Sliced bell peppers with guacamole.

- **Dinner:** Baked cod with quinoa and roasted Brussels sprouts.

- **Dessert:** Matcha green tea chia pudding.

Day 7:

- **Breakfast**: Blueberry and almond butter smoothie.

- **Lunch:** Quinoa-stuffed bell peppers with black beans and corn.

- **Snack:** Edamame beans.

- **Dinner:** Skewers of grilled shrimp served with brown rice and steamed broccoli.

- **Dessert:** Mixed fruit salad with a dollop of Greek yogurt.

Conclusion

In conclusion, "Osteoarthritis-Free Hands: 5-Minute Easy Exercises to Treat Your Own Hand, Wrist, and Fingers" has provided a comprehensive guide to managing hand osteoarthritis and improving hand health. Throughout this book, we have explored the nature of osteoarthritis, its impact on the hands, and the importance of exercise, diet, and additional therapies in alleviating symptoms and enhancing the quality of life.

By understanding hand osteoarthritis's underlying causes and risk factors, readers have gained valuable insights into this condition and its impact on daily life. The signs and symptoms have been elucidated, allowing for early recognition and intervention. The diagnosis process has been demystified, empowering individuals to seek appropriate medical guidance.

The exercises detailed in this book offer targeted relief and rehabilitation for the hands, wrists, and fingers. Through finger taps, wrist rotations, thumb stretches, and more, readers have learned simple yet effective techniques to improve flexibility, reduce pain, and enhance hand function. The additional techniques and therapies explored, such as heat and cold therapy, assistive devices, and lifestyle modifications, provide further support in managing hand osteoarthritis.

We have emphasized the importance of an anti-inflammatory diet, and the included 7-day meal plan offers a practical and delicious way to incorporate nourishing foods that promote joint health and reduce inflammation. Additionally, the exercise tracker bonus provides a means of tracking progress, maintaining consistency, and celebrating achievements.

As readers embrace the exercises, implement lifestyle modifications, and adopt a holistic approach to hand osteoarthritis management, we believe they will experience relief, increased functionality, and improved overall well-being. We hope this book serves as a valuable resource and empowers individuals to take control of their hand health, overcome the limitations of hand osteoarthritis, and live life to the fullest. Together, let us embark on a journey towards osteoarthritis-free hands and a future filled with strength, agility, and joy.

Picture Links

https://pixabay.com/photos/hand-cream-elderly-skin-care-5359396/

https://www.pexels.com/photo/elderly-person-during-drawing-therapy-4566528/

https://www.pexels.com/photo/close-up-photo-of-an-aching-man-holding-his-shoulder-8600449/

https://www.pexels.com/photo/crop-woman-with-clasped-hands-7592507/

https://www.pexels.com/photo/unrecognizable-woman-doing-yoga-exercise-7592362/

WORKOUT TRACKER AND LOG BOOK

Exercise Tracker

To help you stay consistent with your exercise routine and monitor your progress, we are including an exercise tracker as a bonus. This tracker will allow you to record your exercises, track the duration and intensity, and note any changes or improvements you experience over time. By keeping track of your exercises, you can stay motivated, monitor your hand health journey, and celebrate your achievements.

Combining the exercises in this book with an anti-inflammatory diet, you take a comprehensive approach to managing hand osteoarthritis. The 7-day meal plan offers a variety of delicious and nutritious meals to support your hand health and reduce inflammation in the body. The exercise tracker will also help you stay organized and motivated. Remember, consistency and commitment are key to achieving optimal results. Embrace this bonus material, embrace the power of exercise and nutrition, and reclaim a life free from the limitations of hand osteoarthritis.

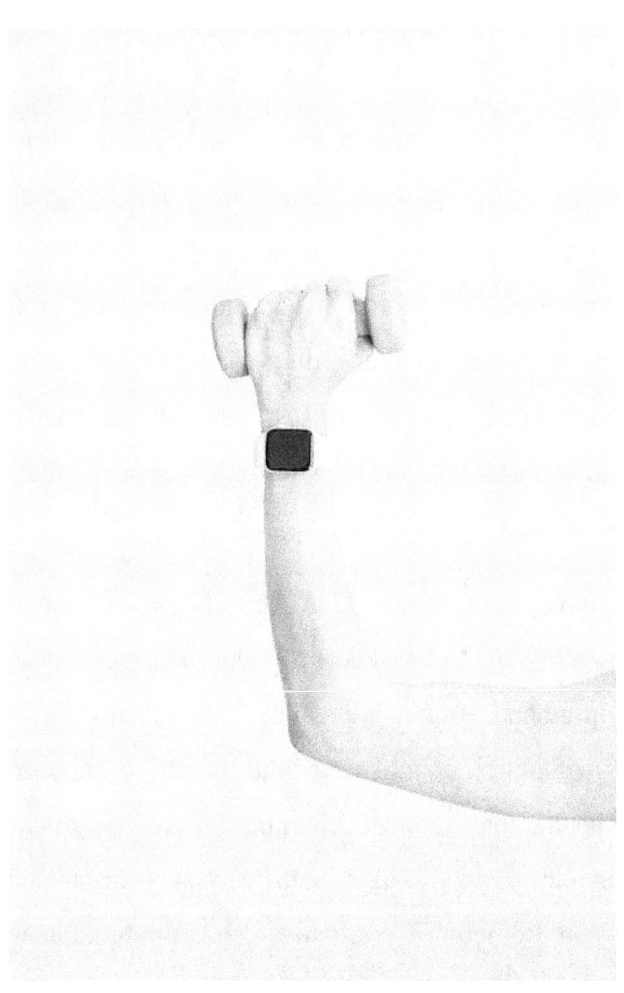

NAME:_____
DATE:_____
TIME START:_____
TIME END:_____

WARM-UP	TIME	NOTES

EXERCISE:	SET 1		SET 2		SET 3		SET 4	
	REPS	WEIGHT	REPS	WEIGHT	REPS	WEIGHT	REPS	WEIGHT

CARDIO:	TIME	DISTANCE	PACE	HR

SUPPLEMENTS & VITAMINS	SERVINGS	QUANTITY

NAME:

DATE:

TIME START:

TIME END:

WARM-UP	TIME	NOTES

EXERCISE:	SET 1		SET 2		SET 3		SET 4	
	REPS	WEIGHT	REPS	WEIGHT	REPS	WEIGHT	REPS	WEIGHT

CARDIO:	TIME	DISTANCE	PACE	HR

SUPPLEMENTS & VITAMINS	SERVINGS	QUANTITY

NAME: _____

DATE: _____

TIME START: _____

TIME END: _____

WARM-UP	TIME	NOTES

EXERCISE:	SET 1		SET 2		SET 3		SET 4	
	REPS	WEIGHT	REPS	WEIGHT	REPS	WEIGHT	REPS	WEIGHT

CARDIO:	TIME	DISTANCE	PACE	HR

SUPPLEMENTS & VITAMINS	SERVINGS	QUANTITY

NAME:

DATE:

TIME START:

TIME END:

WARM-UP	TIME	NOTES

EXERCISE:	SET 1		SET 2		SET 3		SET 4	
	REPS	WEIGHT	REPS	WEIGHT	REPS	WEIGHT	REPS	WEIGHT

CARDIO:	TIME	DISTANCE	PACE	HR

SUPPLEMENTS & VITAMINS	SERVINGS	QUANTITY

NAME: _____

DATE: _____

TIME START: _____

TIME END: _____

WARM-UP	TIME	NOTES

EXERCISE:	SET 1		SET 2		SET 3		SET 4	
	REPS	WEIGHT	REPS	WEIGHT	REPS	WEIGHT	REPS	WEIGHT

CARDIO:	TIME	DISTANCE	PACE	HR

SUPPLEMENTS & VITAMINS	SERVINGS	QUANTITY

NAME:

DATE:

TIME START:

TIME END:

WARM-UP	TIME	NOTES

EXERCISE:	SET 1		SET 2		SET 3		SET 4	
	REPS	WEIGHT	REPS	WEIGHT	REPS	WEIGHT	REPS	WEIGHT

CARDIO:	TIME	DISTANCE	PACE	HR

SUPPLEMENTS & VITAMINS	SERVINGS	QUANTITY

NAME: _____

DATE: _____

TIME START: _____

TIME END: _____

WARM-UP	TIME	NOTES

EXERCISE:	SET 1		SET 2		SET 3		SET 4	
	REPS	WEIGHT	REPS	WEIGHT	REPS	WEIGHT	REPS	WEIGHT

CARDIO:	TIME	DISTANCE	PACE	HR

SUPPLEMENTS & VITAMINS	SERVINGS	QUANTITY

NAME:

DATE:

TIME START:

TIME END:

WARM-UP	TIME	NOTES

EXERCISE:	SET 1		SET 2		SET 3		SET 4	
	REPS	WEIGHT	REPS	WEIGHT	REPS	WEIGHT	REPS	WEIGHT

CARDIO:	TIME	DISTANCE	PACE	HR

SUPPLEMENTS & VITAMINS	SERVINGS	QUANTITY

NAME:

DATE:

TIME START:

TIME END:

WARM-UP	TIME	NOTES

EXERCISE:	SET 1		SET 2		SET 3		SET 4	
	REPS	WEIGHT	REPS	WEIGHT	REPS	WEIGHT	REPS	WEIGHT

CARDIO:	TIME	DISTANCE	PACE	HR

SUPPLEMENTS & VITAMINS	SERVINGS	QUANTITY

NAME:
DATE:
TIME START:
TIME END:

WARM-UP	TIME	NOTES

EXERCISE:	SET 1		SET 2		SET 3		SET 4	
	REPS	WEIGHT	REPS	WEIGHT	REPS	WEIGHT	REPS	WEIGHT

CARDIO:	TIME	DISTANCE	PACE	HR

SUPPLEMENTS & VITAMINS	SERVINGS	QUANTITY